Plant Based Diet For Hepatitis : A Comprehensive Guide To Managing Hepatitis

BY

NANCY BRATTON

Table of Contents:

Chapter Ten: Overcoming Challenges and Sustaining Your Journey

Conclusion

Introduction: The Healing Power of Plants

In a world where health challenges seem to multiply with each passing day, finding effective and sustainable solutions becomes paramount. Hepatitis, a group of viral infections that specifically target the liver, is one such health concern that affects millions of individuals worldwide. The journey towards healing and managing hepatitis begins here, with the understanding that the key to wellness may, surprisingly, be found in the bountiful offerings of nature – the plant-based diet.

The Impact of Hepatitis on Health

Hepatitis is a silent, insidious threat to our health. It strikes without prejudice, affecting people of all ages and backgrounds. Its manifestations can range from mild discomfort to life-threatening conditions, making it a pressing global health issue.

The liver, an unsung hero of the human body, plays a central role in detoxification, metabolism, and digestion. When hepatitis viruses invade this vital organ, they disrupt its normal function. The consequences can be dire, leading to chronic liver diseases, cirrhosis, and even liver cancer.

The Benefits of a Plant-Based Diet

Amidst the medical complexities of hepatitis, there emerges a beacon of hope , the plant-based diet. As our understanding of nutrition and its role in health deepens, we are increasingly discovering the remarkable benefits of embracing plant-based eating patterns.

A plant-based diet is characterized by the abundant consumption of fruits, vegetables, whole grains, legumes, nuts, and seeds, while minimizing or eliminating animal products. It is not merely a diet; it is a lifestyle choice that has the potential to transform health outcomes. The positive impact of a plant-based diet extends far beyond the realms of weight management and cardiovascular health; it reaches the heart of the liver, offering respite to those battling hepatitis.

A plant-based diet revolves around the consumption of foods primarily derived from plant sources, encompassing fruits, vegetables, nuts, seeds, oils, whole grains, legumes, and beans. It doesn't necessitate complete vegetarian or vegan adherence; rather, it emphasizes choosing a larger proportion of your dietary intake from plant-based foods.

Plant-based diets have garnered attention due to their potential health benefits, supported by substantial evidence. Two prominent examples are the Mediterranean diet and vegetarian diet:

Mediterranean Diet: This dietary pattern emphasizes plant-based foods as its foundation but also includes occasional consumption of fish, poultry, eggs, cheese, and yogurt, with limited intake of meats and sweets. Extensive research, including population studies and clinical trials, has shown that the Mediterranean diet can reduce the risk of various health issues, including heart disease, metabolic syndrome, diabetes, certain cancers (such as colon, breast, and prostate cancer), depression, and frailty in older adults. It also enhances mental and physical well-being.

Vegetarian Diet: Vegetarian diets, which exclude meat, have demonstrated multiple health benefits. These include a lower risk of coronary heart disease, high blood pressure, diabetes, and an increased potential for longevity.

Plant-based diets inherently provide all the necessary nutrients, including proteins, fats, carbohydrates, vitamins, and minerals for optimal health. They often excel in fiber and phytonutrient content, which further contribute to their health advantages. However, it's worth noting that some vegans may need to supplement with vitamin B12 to ensure complete nutritional coverage.

To transition towards a plant-based diet, consider these steps:

1. Embrace Vegetables: Incorporate ample vegetables into your meals, aiming to fill half your plate with colorful options. You can also

enjoy vegetables as snacks with dips like hummus or guacamole.

2. Redefine Meat's Role: Reduce meat portions and use them as garnishes rather than the main focus of your meals.

3. Opt for Healthy Fats: Choose healthy fats from sources like olive oil, nuts, seeds, and avocados.

4. Try Vegetarian Meals Weekly: Dedicate at least one night a week to preparing vegetarian meals based on beans, whole grains, and vegetables.

5. Include Whole Grains: Start your day with whole grains such as oatmeal, quinoa, buckwheat, or barley. Add nuts, seeds, and fresh fruits for a nutritious breakfast.

6. Go Green: Incorporate a variety of leafy greens like kale, spinach, and Swiss chard into your daily diet. Experiment with cooking methods like steaming, grilling, braising, or stir-frying to retain their flavor and nutrients.

7. Build Around Salads: Make salads a meal centerpiece by combining greens with various vegetables, fresh herbs, beans, peas, or tofu.

8. Choose Fruits for Dessert: Satisfy your sweet cravings with natural sweetness from fruits like peaches, watermelon, or apples after your meals.

Remember that transitioning to a plant-based diet takes time, but over time, it becomes second nature. Experiment with diverse plant-based ingredients and recipes to maintain variety and enjoyment in your meals while reaping the health benefits of this dietary approach.

Within the pages of this book, we will explore the symbiotic relationship between hepatitis and a plant-based diet. We will delve into the science behind this nutritional approach, unveiling its potential to support liver health, alleviate symptoms, and enhance overall well-being. Through a journey of understanding, practical guidance, and inspiring stories of individuals who have triumphed over hepatitis, we hope to empower you to embark on your own path towards healing.

As you turn the pages that follow, you will discover the healing power of plants, a power that has the capacity to rejuvenate your liver, reinvigorate your health, and redefine your life. Together, let us embark on a transformative journey towards wellness, guided by the principles of a plant-based diet and the promise of a brighter, hepatitis-free future.

Chapter 1: Understanding Hepatitis

Hepatitis is a multifaceted and often enigmatic group of diseases, striking at the very core of our body's detoxification and metabolic powerhouse: the liver. To embark on the journey toward managing hepatitis through a plant-based diet, we must first understand the nuances of this condition. In this chapter, we will delve deep into the world of hepatitis, exploring its types, causes, risk factors, symptoms, and methods of diagnosis.

Types of Hepatitis

Hepatitis is not a single entity but rather a family of viruses, each with its unique characteristics and implications for health. The most common types of hepatitis include:

Hepatitis A: Typically transmitted through contaminated food and water, this acute infection often resolves on its own but can cause severe symptoms.

Hepatitis B: A viral infection that can range from acute to chronic, it is transmitted through contact with infected blood, bodily fluids, or from mother to child during childbirth.

Hepatitis C: Often progressing to chronic infection, it is primarily transmitted through blood-to-blood contact and has been a major concern due to its long-term impact on liver health.

Hepatitis D: This is a rare form of hepatitis that only affects individuals who are already infected with hepatitis B.

Hepatitis E: Similar to hepatitis A, it is usually transmitted through contaminated water and food, and it is generally acute, resolving on its own.

Understanding the specific type of hepatitis you are dealing with is crucial, as it informs the course of treatment and dietary considerations.

Causes and Risk Factors

The origins of hepatitis are diverse, with different viruses and risk factors contributing to its development:

Viral Infections: As mentioned, hepatitis is primarily caused by viral infections, with hepatitis A, B, C, D, and E viruses each having their unique modes of transmission.

Alcohol and Toxins: Excessive alcohol consumption and exposure to certain toxins can also damage the liver and contribute to hepatitis.

Autoimmune Diseases: In some cases, the immune system mistakenly attacks healthy liver cells, leading to autoimmune hepatitis.

Medications: Certain medications, when taken over extended periods or in high doses, can induce drug-induced hepatitis.

Genetic Factors: Genetic predisposition may play a role in some cases, making individuals more susceptible to hepatitis.

Symptoms and Diagnosis

Hepatitis often operates in stealth mode, with many individuals remaining asymptomatic for extended periods. However, when symptoms do manifest, they can range from mild to severe. Common symptoms include:

-Fatigue
- Jaundice (yellowing of the skin and eyes)
- Abdominal pain
- Nausea and vomiting
- Loss of appetite
- Dark urine
- Pale-coloured stools

Timely and accurate diagnosis is critical for effective management. Hepatitis can be diagnosed through blood tests that detect specific viral markers and liver function tests. Imaging studies, such as ultrasound or MRI, may also be employed to assess the liver's condition.

In the following chapters, we will explore the pivotal role that nutrition, particularly a plant-based diet, can play in managing hepatitis. As we journey deeper into the world of plant-based healing, remember that knowledge is your most potent weapon against this silent foe. Armed with a comprehensive understanding of hepatitis, we can now begin to explore the transformative potential of plant-based nutrition for liver health.

Chapter 2: The Role of Nutrition in Hepatitis

The relationship between nutrition and hepatitis is intricate and powerful. In this chapter, we will uncover how the foods we consume profoundly impact the health of our liver, the body's detoxification hub. We will explore how dietary choices influence the progression of hepatitis, emphasising the importance of a balanced diet in mitigating its effects.

Eating Right with Chronic Hepatitis: A Comprehensive Guide

Managing chronic hepatitis can be challenging, but adopting a proper diet is a crucial step in supporting your liver health. The primary goal is to reduce stress on your liver, which is already inflamed due to the condition. Surprisingly, the ideal diet for chronic hepatitis closely aligns with general healthy eating guidelines recommended by the U.S. Department of Agriculture (USDA). A nutritious diet can help you maintain a healthy

weight and support your liver function
effectively.

The Benefits of a Hepatitis Diet:

Chronic hepatitis can lead to symptoms like
fatigue, diarrhea, joint pain, and appetite loss.
As the condition progresses, malnutrition and
muscle loss become more common. Some
individuals also struggle to maintain a healthy
weight. Following dietary guidelines from
nutritional experts, in line with the USDA's
recommendations, can help you sustain energy
levels, preserve muscle mass, and achieve and
maintain a healthy weight.

However, it's important to note that as chronic
hepatitis advances, leading to more significant
liver damage, specific dietary adjustments may
be necessary. For instance, individuals with
decompensated cirrhosis, where extensive liver
scarring occurs, may require a special diet to
accommodate their compromised liver function.

Understanding the Hepatitis Diet:

The essence of a hepatitis diet is rather straightforward. It follows the principles of a balanced, nutrient-dense diet that is generally healthy for everyone. This diet emphasizes consuming a wide variety of foods rich in essential vitamins and minerals while keeping saturated fats, trans fats, excess sodium, excess sugar, and alcohol to a minimum.

What to Eat:

1. Vegetables and Fruits: These provide essential vitamins and minerals and can help you maintain a balanced diet. Leafy greens, in particular, may benefit those managing hepatitis by reducing fatty acid composition in the liver.

2. Grains: Whole grains like brown rice, whole wheat bread, and oats to boost your protein intake and help maintain muscle mass.

3. Protein Foods: Consume an appropriate amount of protein (1 to 1.5 grams per kilogram of body weight) from sources like lentils, beans,

nuts, and tofu to avoid malnutrition and muscle wasting.

4. Coffee:Studies suggest that moderate coffee consumption may reduce the risk of advanced liver scarring in people with chronic hepatitis.

5. Healthy Fats:Replace saturated fats and trans fats with healthy plant-based fats like olive, sunflower, or avocado oils.

What to Avoid:

1. Saturated and Trans Fats:Limit saturated fats from red meat and full-fat dairy, and avoid trans fats found in some processed foods.

2. Excess Sodium:Reduce sodium intake, especially if you have ascites (fluid accumulation in the abdomen).

3. Excess Sugar:Cut back on added sugars, as hepatitis is associated with an increased risk of diabetes.

4. Excess Iron: Some individuals may need to reduce iron-rich foods, but consult your

healthcare provider before making major changes to your iron intake.

5. Alcohol:Completely avoid alcohol, as it can worsen liver damage.

Additional Considerations:

Calories:Ensure you consume an appropriate number of calories daily, working with a healthcare provider or registered dietitian to establish the right target for you.

General Nutrition: People with chronic hepatitis may need to monitor their intake of fat-soluble vitamins and minerals and possibly take physician-prescribed supplements.

Toxins:Minimize exposure to toxins, including unnecessary medicines, pesticides, household chemicals, tobacco, and recreational drugs, as these can harm your liver.

Exercise: Engaging in regular physical activity, according to your energy levels and symptoms, can be beneficial for those with chronic hepatitis.

In conclusion, a hepatitis diet is primarily about adhering to a well-balanced, nutrient-dense eating pattern that aligns with general healthy eating guidelines. While chronic hepatitis may pose challenges, proper nutrition is a powerful tool in supporting your liver health and overall well-being. Collaborate with healthcare professionals and registered dietitians to tailor your diet to your specific needs, and prioritize maintaining a healthy lifestyle to manage your condition effectively.

How Diet Affects Liver Health

The liver is a resilient and multifunctional organ, responsible for processing and detoxifying substances that enter our bodies. To understand how diet affects liver health, we must appreciate the liver's role in metabolism, detoxification, and nutrient storage.

Metabolism: The liver plays a central role in metabolizing carbohydrates, fats, and proteins. The nutrients from our diet are processed by the liver to provide energy and maintain blood sugar levels.

Detoxification: The liver is a natural detoxifier, breaking down and removing toxins, drugs, and waste products from the bloodstream.

Nutrient Storage: It stores essential nutrients, including vitamins and minerals, for later use.

However, when the liver is compromised, as in cases of hepatitis, its ability to perform these functions can be impaired. This is where a well-balanced diet can make a significant difference.

The Importance of a Balanced Diet

A critical aspect of managing liver diseases, such as hepatitis and liver cirrhosis, revolves around crafting a well-balanced and nutritious diet. The liver, a vital organ in our body, plays a central role in metabolism, processing various components from the food we consume.

To comprehend the dietary needs for liver diseases, it's crucial to appreciate the liver's functions. One of its key roles is converting carbohydrates into glycogen, which the body utilises for energy. In a damaged liver, this process is compromised, necessitating an increased carbohydrate intake from the diet to meet energy requirements.

Moreover, a significant portion of the blood from the stomach and intestines carries nutrients to the liver, where they are processed. Proteins are broken down into amino acids, carbohydrates into glucose, and fats into fatty acids. Vitamins and minerals are also essential in these enzymatic reactions that convert food into a usable form. Additionally, the liver serves as a barrier, preventing the entry of harmful bacteria and viruses into our system.

For individuals grappling with liver diseases like hepatitis and cirrhosis, dietary considerations are pivotal. The National Health Service in the UK advises a dietary approach that emphasizes high protein and high carbohydrate intake with moderate fat levels, divided into six to eight meals a day to expedite recovery.

A high protein diet is vital for tissue repair, but fat intake should be restricted due to impaired fat metabolism in the liver. In such cases, Medium-Chain Triglycerides (MCT) oil therapy, commonly derived from edible coconut oil, is recommended.

Patients with cirrhosis often face severe malnutrition and require a high-calorie, high-protein diet. However, the amount of protein must be carefully managed to prevent an excess of ammonia in the blood, which too much protein can cause, or hinder liver healing, which too little protein can lead to. Typically, a diet providing around 2000 kcal, derived from 20-25g of healthy fats, 80-90g of proteins, and 400g of carbohydrates, is suitable.

In cases of ascites, a complication where fluid accumulates in the abdominal cavity due to the liver's failure to synthesise plasma albumin, a low-sodium, high-protein diet is recommended.

When liver function deteriorates to the point of hepatic encephalopathy, patients should be limited to 20g of protein in their diet, primarily sourced from skimmed milk.

Certain foods have demonstrated the ability to strengthen the liver. Methionine and cysteine, found in egg yolks, red peppers, garlic, onions, broccoli, Brussels sprouts, sesame seeds, whole grains, and beans, are sulphur-containing proteins that protect the liver and aid in converting fat-soluble toxins into water-soluble forms for elimination.

Choline, obtained from soybeans, egg yolks, fish, peanuts, cauliflower, lettuce, cabbage, lentils, chickpeas, and brown rice, is essential for fat metabolism. The B-complex vitamins, found in nutritional yeast, sunflower seeds, almonds, peanuts, sesame seeds, and brown rice, play a crucial role in liver health.

Furthermore, vitamin C (in mustard greens, cauliflower, red cabbage, strawberries, papaya, spinach, mangos, peppers, broccoli, and Brussels sprouts) and vitamin E (in almonds, sunflower seeds, walnuts, tomatoes, whole grains, and green leafy vegetables) serve as potent antioxidants to protect and treat a damaged liver.

A balanced diet is a cornerstone of liver health, especially when dealing with hepatitis. Here's why it matters:

Optimal Nutrient Intake: A balanced diet ensures you receive the necessary nutrients your liver needs to function efficiently. These include antioxidants, vitamins, minerals, and amino acids.

Support for Liver Regeneration: Certain nutrients, such as B-complex vitamins and essential amino acids, aid in the repair and regeneration of damaged liver cells.

Weight Management: Maintaining a healthy weight is crucial for managing hepatitis. A balanced diet helps control weight and reduce the risk of fatty liver disease.

Minimising Toxin Exposure: By avoiding highly processed and fried foods, you can reduce the intake of harmful chemicals that can burden the liver.

Reducing Inflammation: Chronic inflammation is a common feature of hepatitis. A diet rich in anti-inflammatory foods can help manage this inflammation.

In summary, maintaining a healthy liver through dietary choices involves consuming small, frequent meals, while avoiding junk food, preservatives, alcohol, and carbonated drinks. Staying well-hydrated with water is essential, provided there is no water retention or ascites. Lastly, it's advised to steer clear of sour fruits like lemons and oranges if you have a liver condition. This comprehensive dietary guidance aims to support individuals in their journey towards managing liver diseases effectively.

Remember that your dietary choices are powerful tools in the fight against hepatitis. By embracing a balanced plant-based diet, you are not only nourishing your body but also offering your liver the support it needs to heal and thrive.

Chapter 3: Plant-Based Diet Basics

In this chapter, we will embark on a journey into the heart of plant-based nutrition. We'll explore what a plant-based diet truly entails, its various forms, and the fundamental principles that underpin its potential to support liver health in the context of hepatitis.

What Is a Plant-Based Diet?

A plant-based diet is a dietary approach that centers around foods derived from plants while limiting or entirely excluding animal products. Unlike strict veganism, which excludes all animal products, a plant-based diet allows for some flexibility and can vary in its degree of plant-focused consumption.

Key components of a plant-based diet include:

Fruits: A rainbow of fruits rich in vitamins, antioxidants, and fiber.

Vegetables: A diverse range of vegetables provides essential nutrients and phytonutrients.

Whole Grains: Nutrient-dense grains like quinoa, brown rice, and oats offer energy and fiber.

Legumes: Beans, lentils, and chickpeas are excellent sources of plant-based protein and fiber.

Nuts and Seeds: These provide healthy fats, protein, and essential minerals.

Plant Oils: Healthier plant-based oils like olive, avocado, and flaxseed oil are used in cooking.

Foods to Include and Avoid

When adopting a plant-based diet for hepatitis management, it's essential to make informed choices about what to include and avoid:

Foods to Include:

- A variety of colourful fruits and vegetables for a wide range of nutrients.
- Quinoa, brown rice, and whole wheat pasta are examples of whole grains.
- Sources of plant-based protein include beans, lentils, tofu, and tempeh.
- Nuts and seeds for healthy fats, protein, and minerals.
- Plant-based dairy alternatives like almond milk or soy yoghourt.
- Healthy plant oils like olive oil for cooking and dressings.
- Herbs and spices for flavour and potential health benefits.

Foods to Limit or Avoid:

- Animal products such as red meat, poultry, dairy, and eggs.
- Highly processed foods, including sugary snacks and fried foods.
- Excessive use of refined oils and trans fats.
- Excessive alcohol consumption.

- High-sugar beverages like soda and sugary fruit juices.

The Versatility of a Plant-Based Diet

One of the remarkable aspects of a plant-based diet is its adaptability. It can take on various forms, allowing individuals to choose a level of commitment that suits their preferences and health goals. Some common variations include:

Vegan: is a stringent dietary choice that refrains from consuming any animal-derived products, focusing solely on plant-based foods.

Vegetarian:A vegetarian diet is characterized by the intentional avoidance of meat products, such as beef, poultry, and seafood. However, it does permit the consumption of other animal-derived foods like dairy products (e.g., milk, cheese, yogurt) and eggs, thereby offering a varied and balanced dietary choice that abstains from meat but allows for these specific animal-based ingredients.

Pescatarian: A diet that includes fish but excludes other meats.

Flexitarian: A flexible approach that occasionally incorporates small amounts of animal products.

Transitioning to a Plant-Based Lifestyle:

Embarking on a plant-based diet isn't merely about what you eat; it's a profound shift in lifestyle that can yield both physical and mental health benefits. The essence of a plant-based diet is simple, it predominantly comprises foods derived from plants, encompassing fruits, vegetables, nuts, seeds, whole grains, and legumes. Unlike a strict vegetarian or vegan diet, a plant-based diet allows for the inclusion of animal products such as poultry, beef, eggs, fish, and dairy, but these should play a secondary role in your nutrient intake. While there's no fixed ratio of plant to animal foods, aiming for at least two-thirds of each meal as plant-based is a sensible starting point. The emphasis lies squarely on plants.

The Health Aspect:

A resounding "yes" echoes when considering the healthiness of a plant-based diet. This dietary choice is characterised by nutrient density, boasting ample fibre, healthy fats, protein, vitamins, and minerals. It's a wholesome approach to eating that can effortlessly meet your nutritional needs.

Who Should Consider a Plant-Based Diet:

The appeal of a plant-based diet is universal, with most adults standing to reap its benefits. Research underscores its potential to prevent and manage chronic diseases while reducing reliance on medications. However, if you grapple with a digestive condition, it's prudent to consult your physician before making dietary alterations.

Navigating the Protein Conundrum:

Shattering the misconception that protein is synonymous with meat is vital. The plant-based realm offers a plethora of excellent protein sources, including tofu, lentils, beans, nuts, nut butters, seeds, and quinoa. It's imperative to remember that dairy, eggs, beef, poultry, and fish can coexist within a plant-based diet; they just shouldn't take center stage in your meals.

Embarking on the Plant-Based Journey:

Initiating a plant-based diet may initially seem daunting, but the key is to take it step by step. Begin by incorporating a variety of fruits and vegetables into every meal. Whole grains like oatmeal, quinoa, farro, brown rice, or whole wheat bread should also have a prominent place. To keep hunger at bay, embrace healthy fats from sources like avocados, nuts, olives, and seeds.

To commence, envision each meal or snack as a composition where two-thirds of it comprises plants, with the remaining one-third designated for animal products like eggs, yogurt, fish, or poultry. As you acclimate to a plant-centric lifestyle, gradually reduce animal product intake to once a day.

Sample Plant-Based Meals:

Breakfast: Savour a bowl of oatmeal crafted with almond milk and garnished with walnuts and berries. Alternatively, relish whole wheat bread crowned with avocado and tomato.

Lunch: Delight in a mixed green salad teeming with avocado, olives, feta cheese, tomatoes, and cucumbers, drizzled with balsamic vinegar and olive oil, paired with a multigrain pita. Alternatively, indulge in a whole-grain wrap filled with hummus, tomatoes, lettuce, onion, and olives, along with an apple.

Snack: Recharge with fresh fruit accompanied by almond butter or a handful of nuts. Alternatively, munch on crisp carrots with a side of ranch dressing.

Dinner:Choose between savoring salmon with quinoa and zucchini roasted to perfection in olive oil and lemon or savoring whole grain pasta intermingled with roasted tomatoes, spinach, garlic, and onion, all enveloped in a rich tomato sauce.

In essence, adopting a plant-based lifestyle is not just a dietary shift; it's an enriching transformation that can profoundly impact your well-being. Embrace the bounty of plant-based foods while maintaining a balanced approach that accommodates your preferences and nutritional needs.

This adaptability makes plant-based nutrition accessible to a wide range of individuals, making it a suitable choice for those seeking to manage hepatitis while still enjoying a variety of foods.

Whether you are taking your first steps into plant-based eating or are already a seasoned practitioner, you will find valuable insights and guidance on your journey toward a healthier, hepatitis-managing diet.

Chapter 4: Nutrients for Liver Health

In this chapter, we embark on a detailed exploration of the essential nutrients that play a pivotal role in supporting liver health within the context of a plant-based diet. Understanding the importance of these nutrients and where to find them in plant-based foods is crucial for effectively managing hepatitis.

Essential Nutrients for Hepatitis

The liver plays a crucial role in maintaining over 500 bodily functions, including blood filtration, glucose storage, and cholesterol regulation. It's our body's natural detoxifier, helping remove harmful substances like alcohol and toxins from the blood. To keep your liver healthy, a well-rounded diet is key, focusing on fruits, vegetables, whole grains, healthy fats, and lean proteins. While some may be tempted by restrictive cleanses, they are unnecessary and often ineffective.

It's important to be mindful of foods high in added sugars and saturated fats, such as soda, sweets, fatty meats, and butter, as excessive consumption can harm liver function over time.

Here's a list of nutrient-dense foods that can support your liver:

1. Cruciferous vegetables like broccoli, cabbage, and cauliflower contain compounds that help neutralize harmful substances in the liver.

2. Dark leafy greens like spinach and kale are linked to a reduced risk of liver disease.

3. Seaweed, rich in antioxidants, can benefit those with non-alcoholic fatty liver disease (NAFLD).

4. Coffee, without added sugars or cream, may slow the progression of liver disease.

5. Almonds, high in vitamin E and unsaturated fats, support cholesterol removal from the liver.

6. Sprouted seeds and microgreens are rich in sulforaphane, which combats fatty liver disease.

7. Garlic contains allicin, supporting liver detoxification and weight loss.

8. Onions, shallots, and leeks may prevent NAFLD, even in the presence of other risk factors.

9. Grapefruit contains antioxidants that protect the liver and reduce inflammation.

10. Eggs provide essential nutrients like choline, crucial for liver metabolism.

11. Artichokes contain cynarin and silymarin, which nourish and protect liver cells.

12. Mushrooms may alleviate liver disease, although more research is needed.

13. Berries, rich in polyphenols, can reduce the risk of NAFLD and fight liver cancer.

14. Apples contain phenolic compounds that combat inflammatory diseases and aid digestion.

15. Beetroot, in various forms, reduces cell damage and inflammation in the liver.

16. Fermented foods like kimchi and sauerkraut, rich in probiotics, help break down cholesterol.

17. Yogurt, another probiotic source, decreases cholesterol and benefits liver health.

18. Flaxseed reduces fatty liver and improves glucose and lipid metabolism.

19. Hemp seeds alleviate fatty liver disease by regulating inflammation and oxidative stress.

20. Chia seeds, rich in omega-3 fatty acids and antioxidants, may treat NAFLD.

21. Coconut oil may have positive effects on liver disease, as seen in rat studies.

22. Avocado oil improves lipid homeostasis and mitochondrial function in the liver.

23. Extra virgin olive oil's antioxidants protect liver function and can be easily incorporated into meals.

24. Ginger reduces fat accumulation in the liver and has anti-inflammatory properties.

25. Oatmeal, a soluble fiber, has protective effects on liver damage and obesity prevention.

26. Cumin supplementation reduces oxidative stress and liver damage in high-fat diet-fed rats.

27. Cardamom decreases liver inflammation and has antioxidant effects.

28. Turmeric's curcumin compounds help manage oxidative stress-induced liver disorders.

29. Fatty fish, like salmon, reduces liver inflammation and fat in NAFLD patients.

30. Tofu and soy foods may lower NAFLD prevalence and improve liver health.

31. Beans and legumes are associated with a reduced risk of NAFLD, making them a convenient addition to various meals.

Incorporating these foods into your diet can contribute to maintaining a healthy liver and overall well-being.

The liver, being a dynamic and resilient organ, relies on a variety of nutrients to maintain its health and function optimally.
These nutrients include:

Vitamin A: Essential for the liver's regeneration and immune function. Find it in sweet potatoes, carrots, and leafy greens.

Vitamin C: A powerful antioxidant that supports liver detoxification. Abundant in citrus fruits, strawberries, and bell peppers.

Vitamin E: Protects liver cells from oxidative damage. Nuts, seeds, and vegetable oils are good sources.

Vitamin K: Supports blood clotting and can be found in kale, spinach, and broccoli.

B Vitamins (B1, B2, B3, B6, B12): Vital for energy metabolism, detoxification, and liver health. Whole grains, legumes, and fortified plant-based foods are rich sources.

Folate: Supports DNA repair and can be found in lentils, spinach, and asparagus.

Iron: Essential for transporting oxygen in the blood. Plant-based sources include tofu, beans, lentils, and fortified cereals.

Selenium: A powerful antioxidant that helps protect the liver. Brazil nuts are particularly high in selenium.

Zinc: Supports immune function and can be found in nuts, seeds, and whole grains.

Omega-3 Fatty Acids: Reduces inflammation and can be obtained from flaxseeds, chia seeds, and walnuts.

Amino Acids: The building blocks of protein, essential for liver repair and regeneration.

Legumes, tofu, and tempeh are excellent sources.

Sources of Nutrients in Plant-Based Foods

Plant-based foods are rich in the essential nutrients required for liver health. Here's where you can find these nutrients:

Fruits and Vegetables: An array of colorful fruits and vegetables provides vitamins A and C, as well as various antioxidants. Berries, citrus fruits, and dark leafy greens are particularly nutrient-dense.

Whole Grains: Whole grains like quinoa, brown rice, and oats are packed with B vitamins and folate.

Legumes: Beans, lentils, and chickpeas are excellent sources of B vitamins, iron, zinc, and amino acids.

Nuts and Seeds: Almonds, chia seeds, and sunflower seeds provide vitamin E, selenium, healthy fats, and zinc.

Plant Oils: Olive oil and flaxseed oil are heart-healthy options rich in vitamin E and omega-3 fatty acids.

Fortified Foods: Many plant-based milk alternatives, cereals, and nutritional yeast are fortified with B vitamins, including B12.

As you embrace a plant-based diet to manage hepatitis, focus on a diverse and well-rounded menu that incorporates these nutrient-rich foods. This will not only provide the necessary vitamins and minerals but also offer a wide spectrum of health benefits beyond liver support.

In the upcoming chapters, we will delve into the practical aspects of creating a balanced plant-based meal plan tailored to liver health, including sample meal plans and recipe ideas. By understanding the role of these nutrients and how to harness them in your diet, you can take proactive steps toward managing hepatitis effectively and enhancing your overall well-being.

Chapter 5: Creating a Plant-Based Meal Plan

In this chapter, we will explore the art of crafting a plant-based meal plan that is not only delicious but also optimally supportive of liver health. We'll delve into the practical aspects of designing well-balanced, nutrient-rich meals, providing you with guidance and sample meal plans to jumpstart your journey.

The Building Blocks of a Plant-Based Meal

To construct a balanced plant-based meal plan for hepatitis management, it's essential to understand the core components that make up a nutritious plate:

Fruits and Vegetables: Ensure that 50% of your meal consists of a vibrant assortment of fruits and vegetables. These foods are rich sources of vital vitamins, minerals, antioxidants, and dietary fiber, all of which are crucial for your health. Strive for diversity in your selection to guarantee a wide range of nutrients that your body needs.

Whole Grains: Dedicate a quarter of your plate to incorporating whole grains such as brown rice, quinoa, or whole wheat pasta. These grains are packed with complex carbohydrates, an abundance of dietary fiber, and essential B vitamins, all of which contribute to a well-rounded and nutritious diet.

Plant-Based Protein: Dedicate another quarter of your plate to plant-based protein sources such as beans, lentils, tofu, tempeh, or seitan. These foods are rich in amino acids, essential for liver repair and overall health.

Healthy Fats: Include small amounts of healthy fats like avocados, nuts, and seeds. These provide essential fatty acids, including omega-3s, which have anti-inflammatory properties.

Herbs and Spices: Incorporate herbs and spices like turmeric, ginger, garlic, and cilantro, which not only add flavor but also offer potential health benefits, including liver support.

Sample Meal Plans

To help you visualize what a plant-based meal plan might look like, here are two sample daily meal plans suitable for hepatitis management:

Sample Meal Plan 1:

Breakfast

For breakfast, savor a hearty bowl of nourishing oatmeal adorned with a vibrant medley of freshly picked berries and a generous sprinkling of finely chopped nuts. Accompany this wholesome delight with a serving of plant-based yogurt, elegantly adorned with a delicate drizzle of golden honey.

Lunch

Treat yourself to a satisfying quinoa salad, brimming with a colorful array of mixed vegetables and protein-packed chickpeas. Elevate the flavors with the zesty allure of a lemon-infused tahini dressing. Complement this culinary masterpiece with slices of ripe avocado, elegantly perched atop a slice of hearty whole-grain toast.

Snack
Carrot and cucumber sticks with hummus

Dinner
Stir-fried tofu with broccoli, bell peppers, and brown rice
Steamed spinach with garlic and olive oil

Snack
A small bowl of mixed nuts and dried fruits

Meal Plan 2:

Breakfast
Whole-grain toast with almond butter and sliced banana
Green smoothie with spinach, banana, and flaxseedsSample

Lunch
Lentil soup with a side of whole-grain crackers
Mixed salad with cherry tomatoes, cucumbers, and a balsamic vinaigrette

Snack
Greek-style plant-based yogurt with a sprinkle
of chia seeds

Dinner
Baked tempeh with roasted sweet potatoes and
steamed asparagus
Quinoa with sautéed kale and garlic

Snack
Sliced apple with a dollop of peanut butter

These sample meal plans showcase the diversity
and deliciousness of plant-based eating while
ensuring a well-rounded intake of nutrients to
support liver health.

Remember that individual dietary needs vary, so
you can tailor these meal plans to your
preferences and nutritional requirements. The
key is to focus on a rich variety of plant-based
foods, ensuring you meet your nutrient needs
while enjoying a satisfying and liver-friendly
diet.

In the upcoming chapters, we will delve deeper
into the specific nutrients and dietary strategies

that can be harnessed within the realm of plant-based nutrition to support liver health and manage hepatitis effectively.

Chapter 6: Managing Hepatitis with Plant-Based Nutrition

In this chapter, we dive into the heart of the matter: how plant-based nutrition can be a powerful tool in managing hepatitis. We'll explore the science behind this approach, detailing its potential to alleviate symptoms, support liver health, and improve overall well-being.

The Science Behind Plant-Based Healing

Plant-based nutrition offers a host of benefits that align with the goals of hepatitis management:

Reduced Inflammation: Chronic inflammation is a hallmark of hepatitis. Plant-based diets are naturally anti-inflammatory, thanks to their rich content of antioxidants, phytonutrients, and healthy fats like omega-3s. These components can help quell inflammation in the liver and throughout the body.

Liver Detoxification: The liver's detoxification capacity relies on specific nutrients found abundantly in plant-based foods, such as B vitamins and antioxidants. A plant-based diet supports the liver's ability to neutralize toxins and promote their elimination from the body.

Weight Management: Maintaining a healthy weight is crucial for hepatitis management. Plant-based diets are often associated with weight loss and the prevention of fatty liver disease, a common complication of hepatitis.

Blood Sugar Control: Plant-based diets are naturally rich in complex carbohydrates and fiber, which help stabilise blood sugar levels. This is particularly important for individuals with hepatitis, as unstable blood sugar can exacerbate symptoms.

Reduced Fat Intake: Excess dietary fat can burden the liver, especially in cases of hepatitis. Plant-based diets tend to be lower in unhealthy saturated fats and cholesterol, which can alleviate this burden.

Numerous individuals with hepatitis have experienced significant improvements in their health by adopting a plant-based diet. While every person's journey is unique, here are some common success stories and case studies:

Reduction in Liver Enzymes: Many individuals have reported a decrease in liver enzyme levels, indicating improved liver function, after transitioning to a plant-based diet.

Weight Loss: Weight loss is a common outcome of adopting a plant-based diet, and shedding excess pounds can reduce the risk of fatty liver disease and improve overall health.

Improved Energy: Plant-based eaters often report increased energy levels and a greater sense of vitality, which can be particularly beneficial for those experiencing fatigue due to hepatitis.

Better Digestion: The high fiber content of plant-based diets can alleviate digestive issues often associated with hepatitis, such as bloating and discomfort.

Enhanced Quality of Life: Beyond the physical benefits, many individuals note an improved quality of life, including reduced stress and a sense of empowerment over their health.

Plant-Based Diet as Part of Comprehensive Care

It's important to emphasize that a plant-based diet should be viewed as a complementary component of hepatitis management, alongside medical treatment and regular check-ups. It is not a substitute for prescribed medications or professional medical advice.

Before making significant dietary changes, it's advisable to consult with a healthcare provider or registered dietitian, especially if you have pre-existing medical conditions or are taking medications.

A hepatitis diet plan is a specialized eating regimen crafted to bolster liver health and assist in the management and recovery of hepatitis, a viral infection that targets the liver. It is essential to understand that while diet alone cannot cure hepatitis, it plays a pivotal role in fostering liver function and mitigating further harm.

The primary objectives of a hepatitis diet are to alleviate the liver's workload, provide essential nutrients for recuperation, and uphold overall liver well-being.

For instance, alcohol is widely recognized as a potent liver-damaging substance, and during a hepatitis infection and recovery phase, alcohol must be entirely abstained from, as it can exacerbate hepatitis symptoms and hinder the healing process.

A comprehensive hepatitis diet plan focuses on several key aspects:

1. Limiting Harmful Substances: Foremost, it restricts the intake of substances known to burden the liver. Alcohol, a prominent liver antagonist, must be strictly avoided. Additionally, fatty and processed foods that can contribute to fatty liver disease and worsen liver

inflammation should be minimized or eliminated.

2. Emphasizing Nutrient-Rich Foods: The diet promotes the consumption of nutrient-dense foods like fruits, vegetables, whole grains, and lean protein sources. Protein, in particular, is vital for liver health, as it aids in the repair and regeneration of liver cells. To accommodate potential difficulties in metabolizing protein, sources like lean meats, poultry, fish, eggs, legumes, and dairy products are recommended.

3. Maintaining Hydration:Proper hydration is crucial for supporting liver function, as it facilitates the removal of toxins and waste products from the body. Drinking a minimum of eight glasses of water per day is advised, though individual requirements may vary based on health conditions.

A hepatitis diet plan is not one-size-fits-all, as individual needs and conditions can differ significantly. Consulting with a healthcare professional or registered dietitian is highly recommended to receive personalized guidance tailored to one's specific situation.

Here is a sample 3-day hepatitis diet plan to offer a general idea of what a hepatitis-friendly diet might entail:

Day 1
Meal 1: Oatmeal with almond milk, topped with berries and sliced almonds. Meal 2: Apple slices with almond butter.
Meal 3: Grilled chicken breast with roasted sweet potato and steamed green beans.
Meal 4: Carrot sticks with hummus.
Meal 5: Baked salmon with quinoa and roasted asparagus.

Day 2
Meal 1: Greek yogurt with sliced banana and granola.
Meal 2: Sliced cucumber with homemade dip.
Meal 3: Chicken wrap with whole wheat tortilla, avocado, tomato, and lettuce.
Meal 4: Orange slices.
Meal 5: Grilled shrimp skewers with a side of brown rice and sautéed spinach.

Day 3

Meal 1: Spinach and mushroom omelette with whole grain toast.
Meal 2: Mixed nuts.
Meal 3: Lentil soup mixed greens salad with tomatoes and cucumber.
Meal 4: Pineapple chunks.
Meal 5: Grilled chicken with roasted sweet potato and steamed broccoli.

Now, let's delve into why a hepatitis diet plan is essential:

1. Promoting Liver Health: The liver plays a critical role in detoxifying the body, metabolising nutrients, and producing essential compounds. A hepatitis diet plan actively supports liver health by providing necessary nutrients and avoiding foods that can worsen inflammation or burden the liver.

2. Inflammation Management:Hepatitis leads to liver inflammation, and certain foods can exacerbate this condition. The diet aims to reduce foods like processed items, high-fat foods, sugary snacks, and alcohol that can contribute to liver inflammation.

3. Meeting Nutritional Needs:Hepatitis can cause reduced appetite, digestive issues, and impaired nutrient absorption, potentially leading to malnutrition. A well-structured diet ensures sufficient intake of vital nutrients, including protein, vitamins, minerals, and antioxidants, supporting overall health, immune function, and liver repair.

4. Symptom Management: Hepatitis symptoms often include fatigue, nausea, and loss of appetite. A thoughtfully designed diet plan can help manage these symptoms, improving overall well-being. This can involve easily digestible foods, smaller and more frequent meals, and avoiding triggers that exacerbate discomfort.

5. Supporting Liver Regeneration: The liver possesses a remarkable capacity for self-regeneration. A hepatitis diet plan supplies essential nutrients like antioxidants and specific amino acids, facilitating liver cell regeneration and aiding the healing process.

6. Managing Weight and Metabolic Health: Hepatitis can influence metabolic processes, including fat metabolism and glucose regulation. The diet plan assists in maintaining a healthy weight, managing insulin levels, and optimizing metabolic health, thus reducing the risk of complications like fatty liver disease and insulin resistance.

7. Enhancing Medication Effectiveness:Some individuals with hepatitis require antiviral medications or other treatments. A balanced diet complements the effectiveness of these medications, enhances tolerability, and optimizes treatment outcomes.

When adhering to a hepatitis diet plan, it is imperative to focus on foods that are gentle on the liver and promote its well-being. This includes a variety of fresh fruits, a diverse array of vegetables, whole grains, lean protein sources, healthy fats, low-fat dairy products, herbal teas, and ample water consumption to aid toxin elimination.

Conversely, certain foods should be avoided or minimized to prevent further strain on the liver and worsened hepatitis symptoms. These include alcohol, fatty and fried foods, processed and packaged items, high-sugar foods and beverages, high-sodium foods, spicy or heavily seasoned foods, and raw or undercooked seafood and meats.

In summary, a hepatitis diet plan is a crucial component of managing hepatitis effectively. By adhering to the dietary recommendations, individuals with hepatitis can reduce liver strain, mitigate inflammation, and foster overall liver health and healing. Remember, a well-balanced diet can significantly contribute to your overall health and well-being, and it's especially vital when dealing with conditions like hepatitis.

In the chapters ahead, we will continue to explore specific aspects of plant-based nutrition for hepatitis management, including recipes, meal planning strategies, and ways to overcome challenges on this journey. By harnessing the power of plant-based nutrition, you can take proactive steps toward better liver health and overall well-being.

Chapter 7: Lifestyle Factors for Hepatitis Management

In this chapter, we broaden the perspective on hepatitis management by examining various lifestyle factors that play a crucial role in supporting liver health. While plant-based nutrition is a cornerstone, a holistic approach encompasses other aspects such as exercise, stress management, and sleep, all of which can contribute to a healthier and more resilient liver.

Exercise and Physical Activity

Regular exercise is a powerful ally in the management of hepatitis. Here's how it benefits liver health:

Weight Management: Exercise helps maintain a healthy weight or promotes weight loss if necessary, reducing the risk of fatty liver disease, a common complication of hepatitis.

Improved Insulin Sensitivity: Physical activity enhances insulin sensitivity, which is essential for those with hepatitis to maintain stable blood sugar levels.

Reduced Liver Fat: Exercise can reduce the accumulation of fat in the liver, a condition known as hepatic steatosis.

Enhanced Immune Function: Exercise can strengthen the immune system, potentially aiding in the body's defence against hepatitis.

Stress Reduction: Physical activity is an effective stress reducer, and managing stress is crucial for overall health.

For individuals with hepatitis, it's important to consult with a healthcare provider before starting a new exercise regimen, especially if there are underlying health concerns.

Stress Management

Stress can exacerbate the symptoms of hepatitis and negatively impact liver health. Effective stress management strategies include:

Mindfulness and Meditation: These practices can reduce stress levels and promote emotional well-being.

Yoga and Tai Chi: Gentle, low-impact exercises that combine physical movement with relaxation techniques can be particularly beneficial.

Breathing Exercises: Simple deep-breathing exercises can calm the nervous system and reduce stress.

Professional Support: Consider consulting a therapist or counsellor for guidance on managing stress and its emotional impact.

Sleep and Hepatitis

Quality sleep is a vital component of liver health and overall well-being:

Regeneration: During sleep, the body undergoes critical repair and regeneration processes, including those related to the liver.

Hormone Balance: Sleep plays a role in hormone regulation, including those that impact appetite and metabolism.

Immune Function: A lack of sleep can weaken the immune system, making it harder for the body to fight infections such as hepatitis.

Mental Health: Adequate sleep is essential for mental health and emotional resilience, particularly when dealing with a chronic condition like hepatitis.

To improve sleep quality, consider adopting healthy sleep habits, such as maintaining a consistent sleep schedule, creating a comfortable sleep environment, and avoiding stimulants like caffeine close to bedtime.

Holistic Health and Hepatitis

A holistic approach to hepatitis management recognizes the interconnectedness of physical, mental, and emotional health. Integrating plant-based nutrition with regular exercise, stress management, and restorative sleep can lead to a more comprehensive and effective strategy for supporting liver health.

In the upcoming chapters, we will provide practical guidance on incorporating these lifestyle factors into your daily routine, along with plant-based recipes and meal plans tailored to hepatitis management. By embracing a holistic approach, you can empower yourself to take control of your health and work towards a brighter, hepatitis-free future.

Chapter 8: Recipes for Liver Health

In this chapter, we embark on a culinary journey, exploring a range of delicious and nutrient-packed plant-based recipes specifically designed to support liver health in the context of hepatitis management. These recipes showcase the versatility of plant-based ingredients while ensuring you receive the essential nutrients your liver needs to thrive.

Plant-Powered Breakfasts

Starting your day with a nutritious breakfast sets the tone for a day of liver-friendly eating. Here are some plant-based breakfast options:

Berry and Green Smoothie: Blend spinach, kale, mixed berries, a banana, and plant-based milk for a nutrient-rich smoothie that's packed with antioxidants, vitamins, and fiber.

Oatmeal with Flax Seeds: Cook oats with almond milk, top with flaxseeds, sliced almonds, and a drizzle of honey for a filling and fiber-rich breakfast.

Avocado Toast: Mash ripe avocado on whole-grain toast and add sliced tomatoes, a sprinkle of nutritional yeast, and a pinch of salt and pepper for a satisfying and heart-healthy meal.

Nourishing Lunch Ideas

Lunch is an excellent opportunity to incorporate a variety of plant-based ingredients to support your liver:

Lentil and Vegetable Soup: Create a hearty soup with lentils, carrots, celery, spinach, and vegetable broth. Season with garlic, turmeric, and cumin for added flavor and health benefits.

Chickpea Salad: Toss chickpeas with diced cucumbers, cherry tomatoes, red onions, and fresh parsley. Drizzle with a lemon-tahini dressing for a protein-packed and refreshing salad.

Quinoa and Mixed Greens Bowl: Combine cooked quinoa with a mix of your favourite greens, roasted sweet potatoes, chickpeas, and a balsamic vinaigrette.

Wholesome Dinner Options

Dinner can be both comforting and nourishing with these plant-based recipes:

Stir-Fried Tofu and Vegetables: Sauté tofu with a medley of colorful bell peppers, broccoli, and snap peas. Season with ginger, garlic, and a soy-sesame sauce. Serve over brown rice or quinoa.

Baked Tempeh with Roasted Vegetables: Marinate tempeh in a flavorful sauce, then bake it alongside a selection of your favorite roasted vegetables like carrots, Brussels sprouts, and sweet potatoes.

Cauliflower and Lentil Curry: Simmer cauliflower and red lentils in a rich tomato-based curry sauce with spices like turmeric, cumin, and coriander. Serve with brown rice or whole-grain bread.

Healthy Snacks and Sides

Nutrient-rich snacks and sides can provide additional support for liver health:

Mixed Nuts and Berries: A handful of mixed nuts (almonds, walnuts, and pistachios) paired with a variety of fresh berries makes for a satisfying and antioxidant-packed snack.

Hummus and Veggie Sticks: Sliced bell peppers, cucumbers, and carrot sticks dipped in hummus are a crunchy and nutritious snack option.

Roasted Chickpeas: Toss chickpeas with olive oil and spices, then roast them in the oven until crispy for a satisfying and protein-rich snack.

These recipes showcase the diverse and delectable possibilities of plant-based cooking while ensuring that you receive the essential nutrients required to support liver health. Remember to adapt these recipes to your dietary preferences and requirements while enjoying the benefits of a liver-friendly diet.

7 days meal plan for hepatitis

Creating a meal plan for hepatitis patients requires a focus on liver-friendly foods that are easy to digest and minimize stress on the liver. This meal plan emphasizes a balanced, low-fat, and nutrient-dense diet. Please consult with a healthcare provider or registered dietitian before making significant dietary changes, especially if you have specific dietary restrictions or medical conditions.

Day 1:

- Breakfast

Oatmeal with sliced bananas and a drizzle of honey.
 A glass of apple juice.

- Lunch

Baked chicken breast (or tofu) with steamed carrots and quinoa.
A mixed greens salad with lemon-tahini dressing.

Snack

Greek yoghurt with a sprinkle of chia seeds.

- Dinner

Baked cod (or a plant-based protein) with roasted asparagus and brown rice.
Steamed broccoli with a squeeze of lemon.

Day 2:

Breakfast:
Start your day with a nutritious and satisfying meal by enjoying a slice of whole-grain toast topped with a modest portion of creamy, ripe avocado spread. The whole-grain toast provides a hearty foundation, rich in fiber and complex carbohydrates, while the avocado spread adds a creamy, flavorful touch, loaded with healthy fats, vitamins, and minerals. This breakfast option ensures you kickstart your morning with a balanced combination of energy and essential nutrients.

Scrambled eggs (or a tofu scramble) with spinach and tomatoes.

Lunch:
For a wholesome midday meal, relish a bowl of hearty lentil soup paired with a side of whole-grain crackers. The lentil soup offers a comforting blend of protein, fiber, and various vitamins, making it an excellent choice for sustaining energy throughout the day. Accompany this with a refreshing cucumber and tomato salad drizzled with a tangy balsamic vinaigrette. The salad not only provides a crisp and hydrating element to your lunch but also contributes an array of vitamins, antioxidants, and essential nutrients. This well-rounded lunch guarantees both satisfaction and nourishment, keeping you energized and content.

Snack
Sliced apple with a dollop of almond butter.

Dinner
Grilled salmon (or a plant-based protein) with sautéed spinach and quinoa.
Steamed green beans with a sprinkle of nutritional yeast.

Day 3:

Breakfast
Smoothie with spinach, frozen berries, almond milk, and a tablespoon of flaxseeds.
Whole-grain toast with almond butter.

Lunch
Chickpea salad with diced cucumbers, red onions, and fresh parsley. Drizzle with lemon-tahini dressing.
Whole-grain pita bread.

Snack
Mixed nuts and dried fruits.

Dinner
Stir-fried tofu with bell peppers, snap peas, and brown rice.
 Steamed asparagus with lemon zest.

Day 4:

Breakfast
Whole-grain cereal with sliced peaches and almond milk.
Plant-based yogurt.

Lunch

Quinoa salad with mixed vegetables, black
beans, and a cilantro-lime dressing.
Sliced avocado on whole-grain toast.

Snack
Sliced cucumber with hummus.

Dinner
Baked sweet potatoes stuffed with black beans,
corn, and diced tomatoes. Steamed broccoli
with a squeeze of lime.

Day 5:

Breakfast
Whole-grain pancakes topped with fresh berries
and a drizzle of maple syrup.
Plant-based yogurt.

Lunch
Spinach and arugula salad with roasted beets,
walnuts, and a balsamic vinaigrette.
 Whole-grain roll.

Snack
 A small bowl of mixed nuts and dried fruits.

Dinner

Stir-fried tempeh with mixed vegetables and brown rice.
Steamed Brussels sprouts with a sprinkle of nutritional yeast.

Day 6:

Breakfast
Smoothie with kale, mango, banana, and almond milk.
Whole-grain toast with almond butter.

Lunch
Lentil and vegetable stew.
 A side of whole-grain crackers.

Snack
 Sliced bell peppers with hummus.

Dinner
Baked cod (or a plant-based protein) with roasted zucchini and quinoa.
Roasted carrots with a dash of olive oil and herbs.

Day 7:

Breakfast

Overnight oats made with oats, chia seeds, almond milk, and topped with mixed berries. Plant-based yogurt.

Lunch

Indulge in a flavorful and wholesome culinary experience with a plate of aromatic chickpea and vegetable curry, thoughtfully presented alongside a bed of nutty, fiber-rich brown rice. This delectable dish offers a symphony of flavors and textures, as the chickpeas infuse the curry with a hearty dose of plant-based protein, while an assortment of vibrant vegetables adds a burst of color, vitamins, and minerals. The rich, fragrant spices in the curry tantalize your taste buds and create a harmonious balance of savory and mildly spicy notes.

Accompanied by brown rice, known for its earthy undertones and nutritional prowess, this meal not only satisfies your palate but also nourishes your body with essential complex carbohydrates. This combination ensures a delightful and health-conscious dining experience, maintaining the original essence of a chickpea and vegetable curry served with brown rice while elevating it to a culinary delight that's both satisfying and nutritious.

A side of cucumber raita.

Snack

A small bowl of mixed nuts and dried fruits is a delightful and nutritious snack option. It usually includes a variety of nuts like almonds, walnuts, cashews, and peanuts, combined with an assortment of dried fruits such as raisins, cranberries, apricots, or dates. This snack is known for its combination of flavors, textures, and health benefits.

Here are some key points about a small bowl of mixed nuts and dried fruits:

1. Nutritional Value:This snack is packed with essential nutrients, including protein, healthy fats, dietary fiber, vitamins, and minerals. Nuts provide healthy fats, protein, and a range of vitamins and minerals, while dried fruits

contribute natural sugars, fiber, and additional vitamins and minerals.

2. Energy Boost:The combination of nuts and dried fruits offers a quick source of energy, making it a great choice for a midday pick-me-up or a healthy snack between meals.

3. Antioxidants:Dried fruits often contain antioxidants, which can help protect your cells from oxidative damage and promote overall well-being.

4.Fiber:Both nuts and dried fruits are good sources of dietary fibre, aiding digestion and helping to keep you feeling full and satisfied.

5. Portion Control:Keep in mind that this snack can be calorie-dense due to the natural fats in nuts and the sugars in dried fruits. Therefore, it's important to practise portion control. A small bowl is a reasonable serving size to avoid excessive calorie intake.

6. Customizable:You can tailor your mix to suit your preferences. Some people like to add

seeds, such as pumpkin or sunflower seeds, for extra crunch and nutrition.

7. Allergies and Dietary Restrictions:Be cautious of allergies or dietary restrictions. Some individuals have nut allergies, so it's important to consider alternatives or omit nuts if necessary.

A small bowl of mixed nuts and dried fruits is a tasty and wholesome snack that can be enjoyed in moderation as part of a balanced diet. It provides a convenient way to incorporate a variety of nutrients into your daily consumption while satisfying your taste buds with a delightful blend of flavours and textures.

Dinner
 Baked sweet potatoes stuffed with black beans, corn, and salsa.
 Steamed spinach with a squeeze of lemon.

Continue to rotate and adapt meals from the previous days, introducing variety through different vegetables, grains, and plant-based protein sources. Consider incorporating more liver-friendly foods like garlic, ginger, turmeric, and leafy greens into your meals. Pay attention to portion sizes, and listen to your body's hunger and fullness cues.

Remember to stay hydrated by drinking plenty of water throughout the day, and limit or avoid alcohol and processed foods. Regularly consult with a healthcare provider or registered dietitian to monitor your liver function and make any necessary adjustments to your meal plan.

Chapter 9: Supplements and Herbs for Liver Support

In this chapter, we delve into the world of supplements and herbs that can complement your plant-based diet in promoting liver health and managing hepatitis. While whole foods are the foundation of a healthy diet, certain supplements and herbs can offer additional support when used thoughtfully and under the guidance of a healthcare provider or registered dietitian.

Recommended Supplements

Before incorporating supplements into your regimen, it's crucial to consult with a healthcare provider or nutrition expert to determine which, if any, are appropriate for your specific needs. Here are some supplements that are commonly considered for liver support:

Vitamin D: Adequate vitamin D levels are essential for overall health, including liver function. If your levels are low, your healthcare provider may recommend supplementation.

Vitamin B12: Since B12 is primarily found in animal products, individuals on strict plant-based diets may benefit from B12 supplements. Maintaining proper B12 levels is crucial for liver health.

Milk Thistle (Silymarin): This herbal supplement is known for its potential liver-protective properties. It may help reduce inflammation and promote liver cell repair.

Turmeric and Curcumin: Turmeric, a spice commonly used in Indian cuisine, contains curcumin, which has anti-inflammatory and antioxidant properties. Curcumin supplements may support liver health.

Omega-3 Fatty Acids: While it's ideal to obtain omega-3s from food sources like flaxseeds and walnuts, supplements can be considered, especially if dietary intake is insufficient.

Herbal Remedies for Liver Support

Herbs have been used for centuries in traditional medicine systems for liver support. Here are a few herbs that have gained attention for their potential benefits:

Milk Thistle: As mentioned earlier, milk thistle (Silymarin) is one of the most well-known herbs for liver support. It's believed to have antioxidant and anti-inflammatory properties.

Dandelion: Dandelion root and leaves are thought to support liver health by promoting bile production and acting as a diuretic to help remove toxins.

Turmeric: Besides its culinary use, turmeric has been valued for its potential anti-inflammatory and liver-protective properties. Curcumin, its active compound, is available in supplement form.

Schisandra: This herb is used in traditional Chinese medicine for its potential liver-protective effects and ability to improve liver function.

Artichoke: Artichoke leaf extract may help improve digestion and liver health by stimulating bile production.

It's essential to exercise caution when considering herbal remedies, as they can interact with medications and have varying effects on individuals. Always consult with a qualified healthcare provider or herbalist before using herbs for liver support, especially if you have underlying health conditions or are taking medications.

Integrating Supplements and Herbs

Supplements and herbs should be viewed as complementary to a balanced plant-based diet and not as standalone treatments for hepatitis. They are most effective when integrated into a holistic approach to liver health that includes proper nutrition, exercise, stress management, and adequate sleep.

Remember that the decision to incorporate supplements or herbs should be made in consultation with a healthcare provider who can assess your individual health needs, monitor your progress, and ensure their safe use as part of your hepatitis management strategy.

Chapter 10: Overcoming Challenges and Sustaining Your Journey

As you embark on the path of managing hepatitis through a plant-based diet and holistic lifestyle changes, it's crucial to recognize that challenges may arise. This chapter provides guidance on addressing common obstacles and offers strategies for sustaining your journey toward better liver health.

Common Challenges

1. Dietary Adjustments: Transitioning to a plant-based diet may be challenging, especially if you're accustomed to a different eating pattern. It can take time to adapt to new flavours and cooking techniques.

Solution: Start gradually, incorporating more plant-based foods into your diet over time. Experiment with different recipes and cuisines to discover what you enjoy most.

2. Social Pressure: Social situations and family gatherings may involve foods that don't align with your dietary choices. Navigating these situations can be tricky.

Solution: Communicate your dietary preferences politely with friends and family, and consider bringing a plant-based dish to share. Focus on the social aspect of gatherings rather than the food.

3. Nutrient Concerns: Ensuring you get all the necessary nutrients on a plant-based diet can be a concern, especially for vitamin B12 and iron.

Solution: Work with a registered dietitian to create a well-balanced meal plan that meets your nutritional needs. Consider supplementation for specific nutrients if recommended by a healthcare provider.

4. Cravings: Cravings for familiar non-plant-based foods can be a challenge.

Solution: Explore plant-based alternatives for your favorite dishes. Craving a burger? Try a plant-based burger. Over time, your taste preferences may adjust.

5. Dining Out: Finding plant-based options at restaurants can be challenging, depending on your location.

Solution: Research restaurants in advance, look for vegan-friendly establishments, or call ahead to inquire about plant-based menu options. Be clear with waitstaff about your dietary preferences.

Sustaining Your Journey

1. Set Realistic Goals: Establish achievable goals for your plant-based journey, whether it's gradually reducing animal products or committing to specific plant-based meals each week.

2. Keep Learning: Stay informed about plant-based nutrition and its benefits for liver health. Continually educate yourself to reinforce your commitment.

3. Seek Support: Connect with others who are on similar journeys. Join online communities or local groups to share experiences, seek advice, and find motivation.

4. Celebrate Progress: Acknowledge and commemorate every achievement, regardless of its size, as each step forward is a testament to your growth and determination.
Recognize the positive changes you've made and the benefits you've experienced.

5. Mindful Eating: Practise mindful eating by savouring your meals, paying attention to hunger and fullness cues, and enjoying the flavours and textures of plant-based foods.

6. Regular Check-Ups: Continue to see your healthcare provider for regular check-ups and liver function tests. Continuously track your advancement and be prepared to refine your strategy as necessary to stay aligned with your goals.

7. Persistence: Understand that setbacks may occur, but persistence is key. If you slip up or

face challenges, remember that each day is a new opportunity to make healthier choices.

8. Celebrate Non-Dietary Wins: Acknowledge the holistic benefits of your journey, such as improved energy, better sleep, reduced stress, and enhanced overall well-being.

By addressing challenges proactively and adopting a patient, persistent approach, you can overcome obstacles and sustain your journey toward better liver health through a plant-based diet and a holistic lifestyle. Keep your goals in mind, stay connected to your motivations, and continue to prioritize your well-being.

Moving Forward with Confidence

Reflecting on Your Journey

Take a moment to reflect on how far you've come. Recognize the positive changes you've made, both in your dietary choices and in your overall well-being. Celebrate your successes, whether they're small or significant, and use them as motivation for the future.

Consider keeping a journal to document your journey, including your goals, challenges, and achievements. Reflecting on your experiences can provide valuable insights and help you stay on track.

Setting Sustainable Goals

As you continue your journey, it's important to set sustainable goals that align with your long-term vision for liver health. Here are some strategies to help you set and achieve these goals:

Prioritise Health: Make health your primary goal, rather than focusing solely on weight or appearance. When health is the driving force, you're more likely to make lasting changes.

Break It Down: Transform your ambitious, long-term objectives into a series of bite-sized, attainable milestones. This approach not only enhances achievability but also mitigates the stress of tackling them head-on."

Monitor Progress: Regularly assess your progress by tracking your dietary choices, exercise routines, and overall well-being.
Adjust Your Goals and Tactics Accordingly Based on This Information.

Stay Adaptable: Be flexible and willing to adapt to changing circumstances. Life can be unpredictable, so having a flexible approach to your health journey is essential.

Seek Professional Guidance: Continue to consult with healthcare providers, registered dietitians, or other experts to ensure you're on the right path and receiving the support you need.

Embracing Lifelong Learning

The journey to better liver health is a lifelong process. Commit to ongoing learning and self-improvement:

Stay Informed: Keep up with the latest research on plant-based nutrition and liver health. This knowledge will empower you to make informed choices.

Experiment and Explore: Continue to experiment with new plant-based recipes, ingredients, and cooking techniques. Embrace the joy of discovery in your culinary journey.

Expand Your Horizons: Explore different aspects of holistic health, such as mindfulness, stress management, and physical fitness. These elements can enhance your overall well-being.

Share Your Knowledge: If you're passionate about plant-based nutrition and its benefits, consider sharing your knowledge and experiences with others. You might inspire someone else to embark on a similar journey.

Building a Support Network

Having a support network can make a significant difference in maintaining your commitment to liver health:

Connect with Like-Minded Individuals: Stay connected with individuals who share your goals and values. Join online communities, attend local events, or form your own support group.

Share Your Journey: Openly discuss your journey with friends and family. They can provide encouragement and understanding, even if they don't share your dietary choices.

Professional Guidance: Continue to seek guidance from healthcare providers, registered dietitians, and other experts who can provide personalised advice and support.

Celebrating Your Health

Ultimately, your journey toward better liver health through a plant-based diet and holistic lifestyle is about nurturing your well-being. Celebrate the positive changes you've made and the vibrant health you've achieved.

Practice Gratitude: Cultivate a sense of gratitude for the nourishing foods, physical activity, and well-being you enjoy.
Expressing gratitude has the power to enhance your drive and overall sense of joy.

Share Your Success: Share your success story with others, whether it's through writing, speaking, or simply sharing your experiences. Your journey can inspire and support others on their paths to better health.

Stay Committed: Remain committed to the principles of a plant-based diet and holistic lifestyle, not just for your liver but for your overall health and longevity.

Your journey doesn't end with this book; it continues with each mindful meal, every moment of self-care, and every choice you make to prioritize your health. With confidence, knowledge, and determination, you can move forward toward a future filled with vitality and well-being, managing hepatitis effectively and nurturing your liver health for years to come.

Conclusion: Your Journey to Vibrant Liver Health

Congratulations on completing this comprehensive guide on managing hepatitis through a plant-based diet and holistic lifestyle. Your dedication to exploring the connection between nutrition, liver health, and overall well-being is a powerful step toward a healthier and more vibrant life.

Throughout this journey, you've gained a deep understanding of how a plant-based diet can positively impact your liver. By nourishing your body with nutrient-rich foods, reducing inflammation, and supporting detoxification, you've taken proactive steps to manage hepatitis effectively. Moreover, you've embraced the holistic approach, recognizing the importance of exercise, stress management, and restorative sleep in supporting your liver's resilience.

As you continue, remember these essential points:

- Knowledge is Empowerment: You now possess valuable knowledge about the role of plant-based nutrition in liver health. Continue to educate yourself and stay informed about the latest research and developments in this field.
- Personalization is Key: Recognize that your journey is unique. Your dietary needs, preferences, and health goals may differ from others. Consult with healthcare professionals and registered dietitians to tailor your approach to your individual needs.
- Sustainability Matters: Sustainability is not only about the environment but also about maintaining a sustainable lifestyle. Make choices that you can maintain in the long term, ensuring that your commitment to liver health remains steadfast.
- Progress, Not Perfection: Perfection is not the goal; progress is. Embrace the journey, including its challenges and

setbacks, as part of your growth toward better liver health.

- A Supportive Network: Lean on the support of friends, family, and like-minded individuals who share your values and goals. Seek guidance and encouragement from professionals who specialise in plant-based nutrition and liver health.

- A Bright Future: Your journey doesn't end here; it's an ongoing process of growth and well-being. As you continue to prioritise liver health through plant-based nutrition and holistic practices, you're shaping a future filled with vitality, resilience, and a deep sense of well-being.

Remember that the path to vibrant liver health is a holistic one, encompassing not only what you eat but how you live. By nurturing your liver and your overall health, you're investing in a future where you can thrive, fully embrace life, and enjoy every moment to the fullest.

We appreciate your willingness to join us on this adventure. We wish you a future filled with vibrant health, happiness, and fulfilment. Continue to make choices that nourish your body, nurture your spirit, and lead you toward a life of well-being and vitality.